ACXION FENTERMINA:

Everything you need to know about

using fentermina to lose weight,

control eating and look under

sixteen

By

Camela Kitten

TABLE OF CONTENT

INTRODUCTION

In 1959, phentermine—a sympathomimetic amine anorectic agent—was first made available as a combined anti-obesity medication. It is sometimes referred to as an atypical amphetamine and shares chemical similarities with amphetamine. Phentermine has been classed as a Schedule IV substance because there has been no evidence that it has an addictive potential (low abuse potential).

In 1959, the FDA gave phentermine

approval for short-term weight management, and in 1960, it was widely utilized. This first medication, which was created by mixing phentermine, fenfluramine, and dexfenfluramine, was withdrawn from the market after many reports of aberrant valves were found in nearly 30% of users.

Later, in 2012, topiramate was added to the list of drugs that may be combined with phentermine to create a new alternative that needed lower doses of the former drug to produce the same results.

Mechanism for weight loss

One of the most effective prescription drugs for weight loss is phentermine. It is used to treat obesity in those who cannot lose weight by exercising and eating well.

Numerous studies have demonstrated that phentermine should only be used by itself to maximize its appetite suppression advantages and reduce the risks of adverse effects, despite the fact that it has historically been used in combination with other weight reduction medications.

As an indirect-acting sympathomimetic, phentermine works by causing and stimulating the lateral hypothalamus' presynaptic vesicles to release the neurotransmitters noradrenaline(norepinephrine) and dopamine. The beta2-adrenergic receptors are stimulated as a result of the rise in noradrenaline levels in the synaptic cleft which may account for its appetite suppressing effects.

Due to the rise in norepinephrine and dopamine levels as well as its indirect impact on serotonin, phentermine is categorized as an indirect sympathomimetic.

According to several findings, phentermine blocks the neuropeptide Y signaling pathway, which is a crucial one for triggering hunger. Since the body is constantly in a state of flight or fight and is focused on the need for energy right away, this combined action suppresses the hunger signal.

Phentermine is grouped under the class of drugs known as anorectics or anorexigenics.

As previously mentioned, it accomplishes this by raising the concentrations of particular neurotransmitters in your brain (dopamine, serotonin, and norepinephrine). Your brain produces more of these neurotransmitters, which reduces your cravings and hunger. However, phentermine should lessen hunger in persons who have trouble sticking to their healthy suggested calorie intake, unlike hCG injections (used to diminish your appetite during a low-calorie phase of the hCG diet). Therefore, using phentermine to skip meals or starve yourself is not advised. Additionally, depriving yourself of food can quickly result in a decrease in the activity of your metabolism, which will slow it down and prevent you from losing additional weight. Phentermine should be added to a well monitored weight loss regimen.

Phentermine reaches its peak levels after three to four hours. According to studies, phentermine generally aids in an additional pound of weight loss per week. The initial weeks of therapy are when weight loss happens at the fastest rate.

USAGE AND DOSAGE

Amphetamines and phentermine share similarities. It activates your brain and neurological system, raising your pulse rate and blood pressure while suppressing your appetite.

Phentermine is used over a short period of time (for a few weeks) for treatment of exogenous obesity in individuals with a body mass index (BMI) of 30 kg/m2 or higher initially, or a BMI of 27 kg/m2 or higher in the presence of additional risk factors (e.g., controlled hypertension, diabetes, hyperlipidemia).

Usual Adult Dose for Obesity:

8mg tablet taken by mouth three times a day 30mins before meal. Some patients may require 4mg(half tablet) three times daily before meals.

15 and 30 mg capsules: 15 or 30 mg are taken by mouth approximately 2 hours after breakfast

37.5 mg capsules and tablets: 37.5

mg taken by mouth once a day before breakfast or 1 to 2 hours after breakfast

Some patients may only need 18.75 mg (one-half tablet) taken by mouth once a day OR 18.75 mg orally twice a day

DOSE INSTRUCTIONS

If you frequently take acxion pills, this time frame shouldn't go above 12 weeks. Never use phentermine in excess of the recommended dosage or for longer than advised.Taking it longer than required will not make it more effective. It is possible that taking more of this drug will have serious, potentially fatal side effects.

A dosage of 30 mg can be taken once daily by adults over the age of 17.

To achieve a satisfactory response with the lowest possible dose, dosage should be personalized.

Due to the potential for sleeplessness, late-night dosing should be avoided.

Do not disregard what the physician advises regarding the quantity of doses and length of Axion treatment (axcion).

Without a prescription, it is not advised to take more medication than is prescribed, and it is against the law to use this medication unless a doctor has prescribed it.

Tablets and capsules are given one to two hours after meals or 30 minutes prior to the first meal.

This diet pill may be given to you by

your doctor in divided doses.

The dosage should be decided by the doctor based on your specific medical needs.

Acxion tablets, commonly referred to as acxion, can be quite helpful for you.

Drug therapy will inspire more confidence with careful use.

Additionally, using this product will aid in weight loss.

It's possible for phentermine to cause addiction. Misuse can result in overdose, addiction, or death. It is against the law to sell or give out this acxion pill without a doctor's recommendation.

If you believe this medication is not working as well as it should be or if you have not lost at least 4 pounds in 4 weeks, call your doctor right away.

Avoid stopping this medication abruptly to avoid unpleasant withdrawal symptoms. To stop using this medication safely, consult your doctor.

If you forgot or missed a dose, take it as soon as you can but if very late in the day skip the dose. Do not take more than one dose each time.

In cases of overdosing, consult your doctor for advice.

SIDE EFFECTS

Common side effects of phentermine include:

itching;

dizziness

headache;

dry mouth;

unpleasant taste;

diarrhea;

constipation;

Insomnia

stomach pain; or

either an increase or reduction in

sex desire.

Serious side effects experience include:
shortness of breath, even with little exertion;
chest ache with a sensation of impending faintness;
swelling in your ankles or feet;
a racing heartbeat or chest fluttering; tremors, feeling restless, trouble sleeping; unusual changes in mood or behavior; or
elevated blood pressure - serious headache, blurry vision, banginging in your neck or ears, agitation, nosebleed.

Most side effects resolve 3-5 days after initiating treatment but if after 5days you are still feeling uneasy, seek medical attention.

Contraindications

Phentermine should not be taken if:
You have cardiovascular disease e.g., arrhythmias, congestive heart failure, coronary artery disease, uncontrolled hypertension, stroke
You are currently using or have recently finished taking monoamine oxidase inhibitors.
You have hyperthyroidism

You have glaucoma

You have a history of drug misuse.

You are pregnant or nursing a baby

You have an allergy to or sensitivity
to other stimulant medications.

Interactions

When combined with phentermine, medications that interact with it may lessen its effects, shorten the duration, exacerbate their side effects, or have no effect at all. There are situations when a drug interaction necessitates stopping the use of one of the drugs, but it is not always the case. The best way to handle drug interactions is to discuss it with your doctor.

Let your doctor know if you are on any other medication before initiating treatment with phentermine.

Other medications for weight reduction (including other prescribed products, over-the-counter remedies, or herbal supplements), antidepressants, antipsychotics, antidiabetic medications, and other central nervous system stimulants may interact with this medication. When phentermine is used with fenfluramine or dexfenfluramine, primary pulmonary hypertension (PPH), a lung illness that frequently results in death, can happen.

Alcohol or taking illegal or recreational drugs should be avoided while taking phentermine.

Use In Pregnancy

A minimal weight gain and no weight loss are currently advised for all pregnant women, including those who are already overweight or obese, due to the mandatory weight gain that takes place in maternal tissues during pregnancy. Weight reduction offers no potential benefits to a pregnant woman. Women who become pregnant while in therapy should be informed of the potential risks to the fetus.

Use in breastfeeding

Given the possibility of major side effects in nursing infants, a choice should be made on whether to stop breastfeeding or to stop taking the medication, taking into account the significance of the medication to the mother.

Use In Liver Impairment

In the case of live injury or disease, no dose adjustment is needed.

Use In Kidney Impairment

In mild to moderate renal impairment: No adjustment is required

In Severe renal impairment (eGFR 15 to 29 mL/min/1.73 m2): Maximum dose: 15 mg/day

ESRD (eGFR less than 15

mL/min/1.73 m2): Its use should be totally avoided

Use In The Elderly

Care should be taken while choosing a dose, typically beginning at the low end of the dosing range. Take into account keeping an eye on renal function as this medication is largely eliminated through the kidneys.

HOW TO MAKE PHENTERMINE MORE EFFECTIVE

Despite the availability of over-the-counter phentermine choices, it is not advised to use this medication for weight loss on your own or without a doctor's prescription. An expert doctor will first evaluate your situation, decide whether or not you are qualified to take phentermine, and provide you with all the information you require regarding the dosage, your advised diet, and an exercise program.

The proper timing of phentermine

use is among the most crucial considerations. Phentermine should be taken once daily, first thing in the morning, on an empty stomach, for the best results. By doing this, you'll ensure that you receive all of its advantages throughout the day and reduce the possibility of adverse effects.

Regularity is another important factor, so make every effort to maintain consistency during your phentermine therapy. Before doing anything on your own after skipping a dosage, talk to your doctor.

Phentermine can considerably

accelerate your weight loss in a short amount of time even though it is not a magic medication and won't melt away your pounds on its own.

Here are ways to make it more effective

- **Establish reasonable expectations:**

It's crucial that you first discuss setting reasonable goals that fall within a healthy weight-loss range with your doctor. Even while it could seem like a simple first step, keep in mind that the scale's reading only represents a small portion of the overall objective concept. To start, we advise you to identify your finish line because knowing it is there and getting closer to it may greatly motivate you to keep moving in that direction. Making your objective simultaneously achievable can stop you from giving up in the middle of the process. Next, you can improve your chances of success by surrounding yourself with people you love and trust who will encourage you and hold you responsible for your actions.

Instead of choosing someone to encourage you with blaming and other destructive strategies, choose someone who can spur you on with their optimism. Ask your doctor for support and professional assistance if you believe this step is out of your reach. Remember to make your goal measurable at the end because only then will you be able to know if you've succeeded. We're not suggesting that you weigh yourself repeatedly throughout the day; instead, use a measuring tape or some of your favorite clothes to see how they fit as the days go by.

- **Consume enough water**

You've probably heard this a million times, but if you've ever consumed more water, you've undoubtedly seen a number of health advantages. Simply simply, drinking adequate water helps your body function at its best. It elevates your mood, feeds your skin, and aids in the body's removal of all the extra water it has been retaining. Usually, the extra water collects in the region around your legs or stomach. It usually results from a poor, high-sodium diet or from not drinking enough water. When taking phentermine and drinking more water at the same time, many experience quick weight loss.

Additionally, one of the most typical phentermine adverse effects, dry mouth, is avoided by drinking enough water while taking it.

- **Have a healthy diet**

People frequently believe that taking phentermine makes it simpler to starve themselves and consume minimal amounts of just about any food. However, we admonish our patients to avoid starving themselves and instead try to develop a positive relationship with food and develop self-control by consuming wholesome portions of nutritionally sound meals. Avoiding foods high in saturated fat, sugar, salt, and preservatives is essential since they cause your body to excrete phentermine more quickly by raising the pH of your urine. However, by consuming foods rich in essential nutrients, you may ensure that your urine has an alkaline pH, which will assist your body remove phentermine gradually.

Once your appetite becomes suppressed, skipping meals could seem appealing, but we strongly advise against doing so. Both your body and metabolism require fuel to operate properly. As previously discussed, many sorts of metabolism failure can swiftly result from starvation and skipping meals.

- **Combine cardio and weight-bearing activities**

Although the prior guidance is

usually more than enough to help you lose weight while taking phentermine, adding cardio and weight-bearing activities can greatly speed up the process and provide a variety of other advantages. You can increase your metabolism and raise your heart rate by engaging in cardio exercises (such running, dancing, aerobics, etc.) a few times per week. This is crucial because phentermine's effectiveness tends to wane over time, and cardio exercises can keep you from developing medication resistance or hitting a plateau in your weight reduction. However, lifting weights results in lean muscles, which in turn help you burn more fat even while you're at rest.

In order to determine which kind of exercise best meets your needs and objectives, we advise speaking with your doctor. If going to the gym is not an option, you can still exercise by walking, hiking, or swimming (which is a great alternative because it doesn't put additional strain on your joints).

- **Make a commitment to a long -term healthy lifestyle**

Despite being an FDA-approved medication, phentermine is only permitted for uses that last no more than 30 consecutive days. Because of this, you should think of it as a helpful tool to get you started on the road to weight loss. However, once you've experienced that initial boost, it's up to you to commit to a long-term healthy lifestyle. You also need to give yourself adequate downtime to recover and get better-quality sleep in addition to maintaining a nutritionally balanced diet and exercising frequently. By doing this, you'll stop those extra pounds from

creeping back on and ensure your
general wellbeing.

CONCLUSION

Here is a summary of all you need to know about phentermine before taking it for weight loss

It's advisable to consult your doctor before deciding to start obesity treatment on phentermine.

Phentermine is not suitable for children below 17years of age.

Give either prior to breakfast or one to two hours after. Do not administer in the late evening as this may result in insomnia. Two doses per day may be beneficial for certain persons.

Various people require different dosages. Take the whole amount of time recommended. Consult your doctor if you notice that you are gaining weight while taking phentermine.

Along with dietary adjustments, physical activity, and behavioral modification as discussed with your doctor, phentermine should be utilized.

If this medication makes you lose your judgment, do not drive or operate machinery.

While taking phentermine, avoid drinking alcohol since it may raise your risk of adverse effects and further impair your judgment.

Phentermine should not be taken concurrently with other weight-loss drugs or supplement.

Only those with an initial BMI of equal to or greater than 30 kg/m2, or those with risk factors for a cardiovascular event at 27 kg/m2, should use this (such as high blood pressure, diabetes, or high cholesterol). Don't give anyone else your phentermine (this is also illegal).

Inform your doctor right away if you experience any new shortness of breath, angina discomfort, fluid retention in the legs or feet, or a decline in your capacity for exercise that is not caused by another condition.

Drug users might seek out phentermine, and dogs or children could die from an accidental overdose. Keep goods out of people's eyes and grasp.

Inform your doctor if you are nursing a baby, pregnant, or planning a pregnancy.

Made in the USA
Middletown, DE
22 November 2022

15590837R00027